BREIANNA L. W. PETTWAY

Medicinal Mushrooms

*Discover the Healing Power of Mushrooms Doctors
Won't Tell You About*

Resources:

OpenAI. (2022). ChatGPT (Version 3.5) [Online AI language model]. Retrieved from https://openai.com/chatgpt Accessed: February 24, 2024

First edition

This book was professionally typeset on Reedsy. Find out more at reedsy.com

Contents

1

Introduction

Ever wondered how nature holds the key to some of our most potent remedies? Welcome to the world of medicinal mushrooms, where ancient wisdom meets modern science in a symbiotic dance of healing. Picture this: deep in the heart of dense forests, amidst the damp earth and whispering leaves, lies a treasure trove of health waiting to be discovered. It's here we find our heroes: Reishi, Lion's Mane, Cordyceps, Turkey Tail, Chaga, and Shiitake – the guardians of vitality, each with its own unique gifts to bestow upon us.

Before we begin this journey of exploration, let's pause for a moment to marvel at the wonder of nature's pharmacy. For centuries, indigenous cultures across the globe have revered mushrooms not just as a source of sustenance, but as sacred allies in the quest for well-being. And now, as modern science unravels the mysteries of these humble fungi, we're beginning to understand just how profound their impact can be.

From boosting immunity to supporting mental health, these remarkable fungi hold the key to unlocking a world of wellness. So, dear reader, strap in as we embark on a voyage through the enchanted realm of medicinal mushrooms – where nature's bounty awaits to nourish body, mind, and soul.

In the hustle and bustle of our modern lives, it's easy to forget the simple truth that lies at the heart of our existence: our connection to nature. Nestled within the embrace of the natural world, there exists powerful healing waiting to be unearthed. Welcome, to the mystical realm of medicinal mushrooms – where ancient wisdom meets cutting-edge science in a dance of renewal and longevity.

Why this book, you might ask? It's simple – because I've witnessed firsthand the transformative power of medicinal mushrooms in my own life and the lives of those I love. I believe and know that these mushrooms hold within them the keys to a life of vibrant health and well-being. And now, it's my honor and privilege to help you unlock the secrets of nature's pharmacy and begin to improve the quality of your life.

So, what can you expect from the pages that lie ahead? Crystal clarity, for one. In this book, we'll dive deep into the world of medicinal mushrooms, exploring their benefits and practical applications for enhancing your quality of life. From bolstering your immune system to balancing your body's natural rhythms, each chapter will illuminate a different facet of the healing power of these extraordinary fungi.

But this book is more than just a compendium of facts and figures – it's a roadmap to a healthier, more vibrant life. As we traverse the terrain of wellness together, you'll not only gain insight into the remarkable properties of medicinal mushrooms but also learn how to integrate them seamlessly into your daily routine. Whether you're a seasoned health enthusiast or just beginning your journey, rest assured that this book has something to offer you.

So, my friend, consider this your invitation to begin a journey of discovery – a journey that promises to unlock the secrets of nature's pharmacy and illuminate the path to an easy mind and energetic body. Are you ready to take the first step? If so, turn the page and let the adventure begin.

2

Boost Immunity

How Medicinal Mushrooms Boost Immunity and Fight Infections

U nderstanding the Immune System and Its Importance
Your immune system is your body's defense mechanism against harmful invaders like bacteria, viruses, and other pathogens. Think of it as your personal army, constantly patrolling and guarding your body to keep you healthy. It's made up of various components, including physical barriers like your skin and mucous membranes, as well as specialized cells and proteins that work together to identify and neutralize threats.

But why is it so important to keep your immune system strong? Well, simply put, a robust immune system is your first line of defense against illness and infection. When your immune system is functioning optimally, it can quickly recognize and eliminate harmful invaders, helping you avoid sickness and recover more quickly when you do get sick.

Moreover, a strong immune system isn't just about fighting off acute infections – it also plays a crucial role in maintaining overall health and well-being. Research has shown that a healthy immune system is linked to lower rates of chronic diseases, faster wound healing, and even improved mental health.

Mushroom Immunomodulators: How Mushrooms Support Immune Health

Now that we've covered the basics of the immune system, let's dive into how medicinal mushrooms can give it a boost. These fungi contain special compounds known as immunomodulators, which help regulate and enhance the function of your immune system.

Beta-glucans, polysaccharides, and other bioactive molecules found in mushrooms act as molecular messengers, signaling your immune cells to ramp up their defenses against potential threats. Essentially, they help your immune system work smarter and more efficiently, enabling it to identify and neutralize pathogens more effectively.

By incorporating medicinal mushrooms into your diet or supplement regimen, you can provide your immune system with the support it needs to function optimally. Whether you're looking to ward off colds and flu or simply want to maintain overall wellness, these natural allies can help bolster your body's defenses and keep you feeling your best.

Reishi: The King of Immune-Boosting Mushrooms

First up, Reishi. This mushroom is a powerhouse for immune support, thanks to its anti-inflammatory properties.

Imagine walking through a serene forest, surrounded by towering trees and dappled sunlight filtering through the canopy. Among the moss-covered logs and fallen leaves, you spot a majestic sight – the Reishi mushroom, also known as the "mushroom of immortality" in ancient Chinese medicine. With its distinctive kidney-shaped cap and glossy, reddish-brown hue, Reishi stands out as a symbol of resilience and vitality in the natural world.

But Reishi's beauty is more than skin deep – it harbors a wealth of health-promoting compounds that have captured the attention of scientists and healers alike. At the heart of its immune-boosting power lies a potent arsenal of bioactive molecules, including beta-glucans, triterpenes, and polysaccharides. These compounds work in harmony to fortify your body's defenses, enhancing the activity of immune cells such as macrophages, natural killer cells, and T-cells.

What sets Reishi apart is its ability to modulate immune responses, striking a delicate balance between activation and suppression as needed. This adaptogenic quality makes it especially valuable in supporting immune health, helping your body mount a swift and effective defense against pathogens while also preventing excessive inflammation and autoimmune reactions.

So, the next time you spot a Reishi mushroom peeking out from the forest floor, take a moment to marvel at its beauty and resilience. And remember, by incorporating Reishi into your daily routine, you're not just nourishing your body – you're harnessing the transformative power of nature to support your immune health and vitality from within.

Turkey Tail: Boosting Immune Resilience

Next, meet Turkey Tail. Its name might be funny, but its ability to boost immune resilience is no joke. It's great for fighting off infections.

Imagine stumbling upon a patch of Turkey Tail mushrooms in the forest – their colorful, fan-shaped caps beckoning you closer. These unassuming fungi are more than just a picturesque sight; they are potent allies in bolstering your immune system.

Turkey Tail mushrooms are rich in bioactive compounds like polysaccharopeptides and beta-glucans, which play a crucial role in enhancing immune function. Scientific research has shown that these compounds stimulate the activity of immune cells, such as natural killer cells and macrophages, helping your body mount a stronger defense against infections.

Studies have also highlighted Turkey Tail's ability to regulate immune responses, preventing excessive inflammation and promoting overall immune resilience. This makes it a valuable addition to your wellness routine, especially during times of increased susceptibility to illnesses.

Shiitake: Strengthening Immune Defense

As you wander through the forest, you may come across clusters of Shiitake mushrooms nestled among the trees – culinary delights with a hidden secret: they're powerhouse immune boosters.

Shiitake mushrooms contain a wealth of immune-supporting compounds, including beta-glucans, polysaccharides, and antioxidants. These bioactive molecules work in tandem to bolster your body's defenses, enhancing the activity of immune cells and promoting overall immune function.

Research has shown that Shiitake mushrooms, in particular, possess potent antiviral and antibacterial properties, making them effective allies in the fight against infections. Additionally,

Shiitake mushrooms have been found to modulate immune responses, helping to regulate inflammation and promote immune resilience.

So, the next time you savor the rich flavors of Shiitake mushrooms in your favorite dish, take a moment to appreciate their role in enhancing your immune defense. With each bite, you're nourishing your body and fortifying your immune system for the journey ahead.

Embracing Mushrooms for Strong Immunity

As we conclude our exploration of the immune-boosting wonders of medicinal mushrooms, it's clear that these fungi hold immense potential for promoting robust health and vitality. From the regal Reishi to the resilient Turkey Tail, and the flavorful Shiitake and Maitake, each mushroom offers a unique pathway to bolstering your body's defenses and supporting overall well-being.

By harnessing the power of these mushrooms, you can empower your immune system to thrive in the face of adversity. Whether you choose to incorporate them into your diet as culinary delights or enjoy them in supplement form, the benefits are undeniable. These natural allies not only enhance immune function but also offer a wealth of additional health benefits which we will talk about later.

So, as you pursue optimal health, remember the wisdom of nature's pharmacy. Embrace the transformative power of medicinal mushrooms and let them be your allies in the quest for true health. With each sip of Reishi tea, each bite of Shiitake stir-fry, you're nourishing your body and fortifying your immune system against whatever challenges may come your way.

In the end, the key to robust immune health lies in embracing the gifts that nature has to offer. So, here's to harnessing the power of mushrooms – may they be your steadfast companions on the path to wellness, today and always.

3

Balancing the Body

Managing Stress, Inflammation, and Chronic Conditions with Medicinal Mushrooms

Welcome to the realm of balance, where medicinal mushrooms serve as potent allies in the quest for holistic wellness. In this chapter, we will jump into the transformative power of mushrooms in managing stress, inflammation, and chronic conditions, offering a roadmap to harmony and well-being.

Reishi: The Master of Adaptogens for Stress Relief

Again, we have Reishi the master of adaptogens – nature's remedy for stress relief. With its potent blend of bioactive compounds, Reishi helps restore balance to the body and mind, promoting resilience in the face of life's challenges. Unmanaged stress can contribute to serious illness and disease so it is so important to learn how to manage and reduce stress.

In the fast-paced world we live in, stress has become an unavoidable part of daily life. Fortunately, nature has provided us with a powerful ally in the form of Reishi mushrooms – revered for their remarkable ability to ease the burden of stress and promote inner calm.

At the core of Reishi's anti-stress properties lies a unique blend of bioactive compounds, including triterpenes, polysaccharides, and antioxidants. These potent molecules work synergistically to soothe the nervous system and modulate the body's stress response, helping to restore balance and harmony in times of tension.

Research has shown that Reishi contains adaptogenic compounds that help regulate the production of stress hormones like cortisol, allowing the body to better adapt to and cope with the demands of daily life. By reducing the physiological and psychological effects of stress, Reishi can help alleviate symptoms of anxiety, improve mood, and promote a sense of overall well-being.

Reishi's calming effects extend beyond the immediate moment – regular consumption of Reishi has been linked to long-term improvements in stress resilience and emotional stability. By incorporating Reishi into your daily routine, you can cultivate a greater sense of calm and resilience, enabling you to navigate life's challenges with grace and ease.

Chaga: Potent Antioxidant Protection for Fighting Inflammation and Disease

Chaga, scientifically known as Inonotus obliquus, presents a distinctive and visually striking appearance. Its exterior resembles a rough, charcoal-like crust, often with deep, irregular ridges and crevices. Despite its rugged exterior, Chaga's interior reveals a vibrant orange or rusty-brown core when broken open, contrasting starkly with its outer surface. Encountering

Chaga in the wild evokes a sense of ancient wisdom and resilience, as this unique fungus thrives in harsh and remote landscapes, symbolizing the untamed beauty of nature's bounty.

Chaga is a strong source of antioxidant protection against inflammation and disease. Bursting with potent phytonutrients, Chaga helps quell inflammation and oxidative stress, offering a shield of defense for your body's delicate balance.

At the heart of Chaga's health-promoting properties lies its exceptionally high concentration of antioxidants, including polyphenols, flavonoids, and melanin. These powerful molecules help neutralize harmful free radicals in the body, preventing oxidative damage to cells and tissues and reducing the risk of chronic inflammation and disease.

Research has shown that Chaga's antioxidant-rich profile confers a myriad of health benefits, from boosting immune function to supporting cardiovascular health and even reducing the risk of certain cancers. Additionally, Chaga has been found to possess anti-inflammatory properties, which can further support its role in combating chronic inflammation and associated conditions.

As you can see, Chaga's immune-modulating effects make it a valuable ally in promoting overall wellness and resilience. By enhancing the activity of immune cells and promoting a balanced immune response, Chaga helps fortify the body's defenses against infections and diseases, ensuring optimal health and vitality.

Cordyceps: Energizing the Body and Balancing Stress Responses

Meet Cordyceps – nature's energizing tonic and master of

harmonizing stress responses. Originating from high-altitude regions like the Himalayas, Cordyceps has long been revered for its ability to invigorate the body and promote resilience in the face of life's challenges. It is characterized by its elongated, slender stalk that emerges from the earth. Atop this stem sits a bulbous, club-shaped fruiting body, often adorned with intricate patterns or textures.

What sets Cordyceps apart is its unique blend of nutrients and adaptogenic compounds, including cordycepin, polysaccharides, and amino acids. These bioactive molecules work together to enhance mitochondrial function, the powerhouse of your cells, resulting in increased energy production and improved stamina.

But Cordyceps' benefits extend beyond providing stamina – it also plays a crucial role in balancing the body's stress responses. Research has shown that Cordyceps contains adaptogenic compounds that help regulate the production of stress hormones like cortisol, promoting a sense of calm and stability in times of tension. This is an amazing tool to have in your belt because high cortisol levels lead to an array of negative side effects like fatigue, headaches, weight gain and intestinal issues.

Furthermore, Cordyceps' ability to support oxygen utilization and circulation makes it especially valuable for athletes and active individuals looking to enhance performance and recovery. By improving oxygen delivery to cells and tissues, Cordyceps helps optimize physical endurance and reduce fatigue, enabling you to push your limits and achieve peak performance.

Turkey Tail: Restoring Balance in Your Gut Microbiome

Turkey Tail, with its vibrant colors and unique fan-shaped appearance, is not only a sight to behold but also a source of many health benefits, including restoring balance in your gut microbiome. This humble mushroom contains a wealth of bioactive compounds, including polysaccharides and prebiotics, that work hand in hand to support digestive health and promote a harmonious gut microbiome.

Research has shown that Turkey Tail possesses potent prebiotic properties, meaning it provides nourishment to beneficial bacteria in the gut, helping them thrive and maintain a healthy balance. By fostering the growth of beneficial bacteria, Turkey Tail contributes to improved digestion, nutrient absorption, and overall gut health.

But Turkey Tail's benefits extend beyond the digestive system – it also holds promise in the realm of cancer prevention and treatment. Studies have shown that Turkey Tail contains compounds known as polysaccharopeptides, which have been found to stimulate the activity of immune cells and enhance the body's natural defenses against cancer cells.

Achieving Balance with Mushroom Medicine

Is it not evident that these remarkable Mushrooms offer a pathway to achieving balance and better health in our lives. From Reishi's calming embrace to Chaga's protective shield, Cordyceps' invigorating energy, and Turkey Tail's gut-nourishing properties, each mushroom brings its own unique blend of benefits to the table.

By embracing mushroom medicine, we empower ourselves to nurture our bodies and minds in profound ways. Whether seeking relief from stress, inflammation, or chronic conditions, or simply striving to support overall well-being, medicinal mushrooms offer a natural and holistic approach to health and vitality.

4

Support Mental Health

Harnessing the power of Mushrooms for mental well being

Mental Health and Mushrooms
Welcome to the crossroads of mental health and mushroom medicine, where the healing forces of nature intersect with the intricacies of the human mind. In this chapter, we will explore how medicinal mushrooms can profoundly impact mental well-being. From ancient traditions to modern science, mushrooms have been revered for their potential to support cognitive function, emotional balance, and overall mental wellness. As we delve deeper into this fascinating realm, we'll uncover the unique properties of mushrooms that make them invaluable allies in the quest for a healthy mind and spirit. So, join me in uncovering the transformative potential of mushroom medicine in promoting mental health and emotional vitality.

Lion's Mane: Nurturing Cognitive Health and Emotional

Well-being

Lion's Mane, scientifically known as Hericium erinaceus, presents a captivating physical appearance reminiscent of its namesake. This unique mushroom species boasts a strikingly shaggy and cascading structure, resembling the flowing mane of a lion.

This is a mushroom revered for its remarkable capacity to nurture cognitive health and emotional well-being. With its distinctive blend of bioactive compounds, Lion's Mane emerges as a potent ally in supporting mental clarity, memory function, and emotional resilience. Delving into the depths of Lion's Mane, we unearth its profound impact on enhancing cognitive abilities and fostering emotional well-being.

Research into Lion's Mane has revealed its ability to promote cognitive function and memory support. Studies suggest that Lion's Mane contains compounds known as hericenones and erinacines, which stimulate the production of nerve growth factor (NGF) in the brain. This essential protein plays a vital role in the growth, maintenance, and repair of neurons, thereby enhancing synaptic plasticity and cognitive function. By promoting the growth of new brain cells and strengthening neural connections, Lion's Mane may help improve memory retention, learning ability, and overall cognitive performance.

Lion's Mane has also been associated with bolstering emotional resilience and mental well-being. Research indicates that Lion's Mane possesses antidepressant and anxiolytic properties, meaning it may help alleviate symptoms of depression and anxiety. By modulating neurotransmitter levels and reducing stress hormone secretion, Lion's Mane promotes a sense of calmness and emotional stability, fostering resilience in the face of life's challenges.

Reishi: Balancing Mood and Promoting Relaxation

Reishi, a mushroom renowned for its ability to balance mood and promote relaxation. With its rich array of bioactive compounds, Reishi emerges as a gentle yet powerful ally in fostering emotional well-being and mental tranquility as well as restoring emotional equilibrium and promoting a sense of calmness.

Research into Reishi's therapeutic properties has revealed its capacity to modulate mood and alleviate symptoms of stress and anxiety. Studies suggest that Reishi contains adaptogenic compounds that help regulate the body's stress response, reducing levels of cortisol and promoting a state of relaxation. By calming the nervous system and soothing frazzled nerves, Reishi offers a natural remedy for alleviating feelings of tension and promoting emotional balance.

Additionally, Reishi has been associated with enhancing mood and promoting feelings of well-being. Research indicates that Reishi contains compounds that stimulate the production of neurotransmitters like serotonin and dopamine, which play key roles in regulating mood and promoting feelings of happiness and contentment. By increasing levels of these "feel-good" chemicals in the brain, Reishi may help lift the spirits and alleviate symptoms of depression and low mood.

Cordyceps: Energizing the Mind and Elevating Mood

Cordyceps is the energizing elixir renowned for its ability to uplift the mind and elevate mood. Beyond its well-known revitalizing effects on physical energy, Cordyceps also holds remarkable benefits for mental well-being. Through its unique mechanisms of action, Cordyceps enhances cognitive function and mental clarity while simultaneously combating fatigue and enhancing mood.

Research into Cordyceps' cognitive-enhancing properties has revealed its ability to improve oxygen utilization and circulation in the brain. By optimizing blood flow and nutrient delivery to brain cells, Cordyceps promotes enhanced cognitive function, including improved memory, focus, and mental clarity. Additionally, Cordyceps' adaptogenic properties help combat mental fatigue and support sustained mental performance, making it a valuable ally for maintaining peak cognitive function throughout the day.

Cordyceps has also been associated with mood-elevating effects, thanks to its ability to modulate neurotransmitter levels and promote a balanced mood. Studies suggest that Cordyceps may increase levels of dopamine and serotonin, two neurotransmitters closely linked to mood regulation and feelings of happiness and well-being. By enhancing neurotransmitter function, Cordyceps helps promote a positive outlook and emotional resilience, even in the face of stress and adversity.

Turkey Tail: Supporting Emotional Balance

Turkey Tail, renowned for its myriad health benefits, extends its therapeutic prowess to the realm of emotional balance, offering significant support for mental well-being. Abundant in polysaccharides and an array of bioactive compounds, Turkey Tail emerges as a natural ally in nurturing emotional resilience and stability.

According to research, the polysaccharides present in Turkey Tail possess immune-modulating properties that extend to the realm of emotions. By regulating the body's stress response, Turkey Tail helps mitigate the physiological effects of stress, such as elevated cortisol levels, which can disrupt emotional equilibrium. This modulation of stress hormones contributes to a more balanced mood and greater emotional resilience.

Furthermore, Turkey Tail's impact on mental health is underscored by its influence on neurotransmitter levels and mood regulation. Studies suggest that certain compounds in Turkey Tail may modulate neurotransmitter activity, including serotonin and dopamine, which play pivotal roles in mood regulation and emotional well-being. By promoting optimal neurotransmitter function, Turkey Tail supports a positive mood and enhances overall emotional stability.

Moreover, the gut-brain connection highlights the significance of immune health in shaping emotional well-being. As an integral part of the gut microbiome, Turkey Tail's immune-supporting properties indirectly contribute to mental health by maintaining gut health and supporting the gut-brain axis. A healthy gut microbiome is associated with improved mood regulation and reduced risk of mental health disorders, further emphasizing the importance of Turkey Tail in promoting emotional balance.

Empowering Mental Wellness with Mushroom Medicine

From Lion's Mane's cognitive-enhancing properties to Reishi's calming influence, Cordyceps' energizing effects, and Turkey Tail's support for emotional balance, each mushroom offers a unique pathway to nurturing mental health and wellness.

By harnessing the power of mushroom medicine, we empower ourselves to cultivate a state of holistic well-being that encompasses both mind and body. Through their diverse array of bioactive compounds and therapeutic properties, mushrooms provide a natural and effective means of supporting cognitive function, emotional resilience, and overall mental wellness.

Whether you're seeking to sharpen your mental acuity, find inner peace, or enhance emotional resilience, mushroom medicine offers a gentle yet potent ally in the quest for mental wellness.

5

Integrating Medicinal Mushrooms into Your Wellness Routine

Recipes, Supplements, and Lifestyle Tips

Welcome to the culmination of our exploration into integrating medicinal mushrooms into your daily wellness routine. It is one thing to know what these mushrooms can do for you, but it is something entirely to incorporate them into your daily life in small ways that will greatly benefit you in the long run. Medicinal mushrooms can be seamlessly incorporated into your life for holistic well-being. From culinary delights to convenient supplements and mindful lifestyle practices, we delve into the multifaceted approaches to harnessing the power of mushrooms for optimal health.

Understanding the Versatility of Medicinal Mushrooms

Before delving into practical applications, it's essential to grasp the multifaceted nature of medicinal mushrooms. Each mushroom species offers a unique blend of flavors, textures, and therapeutic properties, making them versatile additions to any wellness routine. From the earthy richness of Reishi to the savory umami of Shiitake, medicinal mushrooms encompass a diverse range of tastes and aromas that can enhance a variety of culinary creations. Furthermore, beyond their culinary appeal, medicinal mushrooms boast an array of health-promoting compounds, including polysaccharides, terpenoids, and antioxidants, which contribute to their therapeutic benefits. By understanding the nuances of each mushroom species, individuals can unlock their full potential for promoting overall health and well-being.

Culinary Creations: Infusing Mushrooms into Everyday Recipes

Prepare to embark on a culinary journey where medicinal mushrooms take center stage, elevating everyday recipes to new heights of flavor and nutrition. Incorporating medicinal mushrooms into your cooking not only adds depth and richness to dishes but also enhances their health-promoting properties. Below are some delicious recipes featuring different medicinal mushrooms to incorporate your cooking:

Reishi Mushroom Broth

Ingredients:

- 4 cups water
- 1 ounce dried Reishi mushrooms
- 1 onion, chopped
- 2 cloves garlic, minced
- 1-inch piece of ginger, sliced
- Salt and pepper to taste

Instructions:

- In a large pot, bring water to a boil.
- Add dried Reishi mushrooms, onion, garlic, and ginger to the pot.
- Reduce heat and let simmer for 30-40 minutes, allowing the flavors to meld.
- Season with salt and pepper to taste.
- Strain the broth and discard solids.
- Serve hot as a nourishing broth or use as a base for soups and stews.

Shiitake Mushroom Stir-Fry

Ingredients:

- 8 ounces Shiitake mushrooms, stems removed and sliced
- 2 tablespoons soy sauce
- 1 tablespoon sesame oil
- 2 cloves garlic, minced
- 1-inch piece of ginger, grated
- 1 bell pepper, sliced
- 1 cup snap peas
- Cooked rice or noodles, for serving
- Sesame seeds and green onions, for garnish

Instructions:

- Heat sesame oil in a large skillet or wok over medium heat.
- Add minced garlic and grated ginger to the skillet and sauté

for 1-2 minutes until fragrant.
- Add sliced Shiitake mushrooms to the skillet and cook until golden brown, about 5-7 minutes.
- Stir in soy sauce, bell pepper, and snap peas, and cook for an additional 3-4 minutes until vegetables are tender-crisp.
- Serve the stir-fry over cooked rice or noodles, garnished with sesame seeds and green onions.

Lion's Mane Mushroom Tacos

Ingredients:

- 8 ounces Lion's Mane mushrooms, sliced
- 2 tablespoons olive oil
- 1 teaspoon chili powder
- 1/2 teaspoon cumin
- Salt and pepper to taste
- 8 small corn tortillas
- Toppings: avocado, salsa, cilantro, lime wedges

Instructions:

- Heat olive oil in a skillet over medium heat.
- Add sliced Lion's Mane mushrooms to the skillet and season with chili powder, cumin, salt, and pepper.
- Cook mushrooms for 5-7 minutes until tender and lightly browned.
- Warm corn tortillas in a separate skillet or in the oven.
- Assemble tacos with cooked mushrooms and desired toppings such as sliced avocado, salsa, cilantro, and a squeeze

of lime juice.
- Serve hot and enjoy the flavorful and nutritious tacos.

Cordyceps Chicken Stir-Fry

Ingredients:

- 1 lb chicken breast, thinly sliced
- 4 oz dried Cordyceps militaris mushrooms
- 2 tablespoons soy sauce
- 1 tablespoon oyster sauce
- 1 tablespoon sesame oil
- 2 cloves garlic, minced
- 1-inch piece of ginger, grated
- 2 cups broccoli florets
- 1 red bell pepper, sliced
- Cooked rice or noodles, for serving
- Green onions, for garnish

Instructions:

- Soak dried Cordyceps mushrooms in hot water for 20-30 minutes until softened. Drain and set aside.
- In a bowl, marinate sliced chicken breast with soy sauce and oyster sauce for 15-20 minutes.
- Heat sesame oil in a large skillet or wok over medium-high heat.
- Add minced garlic and grated ginger to the skillet and sauté for 1-2 minutes until fragrant.
- Add marinated chicken to the skillet and cook until

browned and cooked through, about 5-7 minutes.
- Stir in soaked Cordyceps mushrooms, broccoli florets, and sliced bell pepper, and cook for an additional 3-4 minutes until vegetables are tender-crisp.
- Serve the stir-fry over cooked rice or noodles, garnished with green onions.

Chaga Chocolate Smoothie

Ingredients:

- 1 cup almond milk (or any milk of choice)
- 1 ripe banana
- 1 tablespoon cocoa powder
- 1 tablespoon honey or maple syrup
- 1 teaspoon Chaga mushroom powder
- 1/2 teaspoon vanilla extract
- Ice cubes, as needed

Instructions:

- In a blender, combine almond milk, ripe banana, cocoa powder, honey or maple syrup, Chaga mushroom powder, and vanilla extract.
- Add ice cubes to the blender for a thicker consistency, if desired.
- Blend until smooth and creamy.
- Pour the Chaga chocolate smoothie into glasses and serve immediately.

Turkey Tail Immune-Boosting Soup

Ingredients:

- 8 cups chicken or vegetable broth
- 4 oz dried Turkey Tail mushrooms
- 2 carrots, diced
- 2 celery stalks, diced
- 1 onion, diced
- 3 cloves garlic, minced
- 1 tablespoon olive oil
- Salt and pepper to taste
- Fresh parsley, for garnish

Instructions:

- In a large pot, heat olive oil over medium heat.
- Add diced onion and minced garlic to the pot and sauté until softened and fragrant, about 5 minutes.
- Add diced carrots and celery to the pot and cook for an additional 3-4 minutes.
- Pour in chicken or vegetable broth and bring to a simmer.
- Add dried Turkey Tail mushrooms to the pot and simmer for 20-30 minutes until mushrooms are tender.
- Season the soup with salt and pepper to taste.
- Ladle the Turkey Tail immune-boosting soup into bowls, garnish with fresh parsley, and serve hot.

These recipes showcase just a few of the many ways you can incorporate medicinal mushrooms into your everyday cooking, infusing your meals with both delicious flavors and health-promoting benefits. Experiment with different mushroom varieties and culinary techniques to discover your favorite mushroom-infused dishes.

Mushroom Supplements and Tinctures: Choosing the Right Products for Your Needs

When it comes to incorporating medicinal mushrooms into your wellness routine, supplements and tinctures offer convenient and concentrated forms of mushroom extracts. However, with a plethora of products available on the market, selecting the right one can be overwhelming. Here are some key factors to consider when choosing mushroom supplements and tinctures to meet your individual needs:

Quality and Purity:

- Look for supplements and tinctures made from high-quality, organic mushrooms sourced from reputable suppliers. Ensure that the products undergo rigorous testing for purity, potency, and contaminants to guarantee safety and efficacy.

Extraction Method:

- Different extraction methods can affect the bioavailability and effectiveness of mushroom supplements and tinctures. Choose products that utilize extraction techniques such as hot water extraction or dual extraction (combining hot water and alcohol extraction) to maximize the extraction of bioactive compounds from the mushrooms.

Mushroom Species:

- Consider your specific health goals and choose mushroom supplements or tinctures that contain the mushroom species best suited to address your needs. As we have found, Reishi, Lion's Mane, Cordyceps, Chaga, Turkey Tail, and Shiitake, all offer unique health-promoting properties.

Dosage and Concentration:

- Pay attention to the dosage and concentration of active ingredients in mushroom supplements and tinctures. Opt for products with standardized extracts or clear dosage recommendations to ensure consistency and efficacy.

Formulation and Additional Ingredients:

- Some mushroom supplements and tinctures may contain additional ingredients or synergistic blends designed to enhance their effects. Consider whether you prefer standalone mushroom extracts or formulations that include complementary herbs, vitamins, or minerals to support specific health concerns.

Reputation and Reviews:

- Research the reputation of the brand and read customer reviews to gauge the effectiveness and quality of the mushroom supplements and tinctures. Look for brands with positive feedback and transparent manufacturing practices.

Consultation with Healthcare Professional:

- If you have any underlying health conditions or are taking medications, consult with a healthcare professional before adding mushroom supplements or tinctures to your wellness routine. They can provide personalized recommendations based on your individual health status and medical history.

By considering these factors and conducting thorough research, you can confidently select mushroom supplements and tinctures that align with your health goals and preferences. Whether you're looking to boost immunity, support cognitive function, or enhance overall vitality, choosing the right products can help you harness the full potential of medicinal mushrooms for your life.

Lifestyle Tips for Maximizing Mushroom Benefits

Beyond the plate and pill, lifestyle factors play a significant role in maximizing the benefits of medicinal mushrooms. From stress management techniques to sleep hygiene practices and mindful movement, incorporating holistic wellness practices into your daily routine can amplify the effects of mushrooms in your daily life. In this section, we offer lifestyle tips for optimizing mushroom benefits and enhancing holistic well-being.

Stress Management:

- Practice stress-reduction techniques such as meditation, deep breathing exercises, yoga, or tai chi to promote relaxation and reduce cortisol levels, which can inhibit immune function and contribute to inflammation.

Quality Sleep:

- Prioritize quality sleep by establishing a regular sleep schedule, creating a calming bedtime routine, and optimizing your sleep environment. Adequate rest supports immune function, cognitive health, and overall well-being.

Balanced Nutrition:

- Maintain a balanced diet rich in whole foods, fruits, vegetables, lean proteins, and healthy fats to provide essential nutrients and support optimal immune function and overall health.

Regular Exercise:

- Engage in regular physical activity, such as walking, jogging, cycling, or strength training, to boost circulation, improve mood, and support immune function. Aim for at least 30 minutes of moderate-intensity exercise most days of the week.

Mindfulness and Meditation:

- Cultivate mindfulness through meditation, mindfulness practices, or spending time in nature to reduce stress, enhance emotional well-being, and foster a deeper connection with yourself and the world around you.

Social Connection:

- Foster meaningful connections with friends, family, and community members to promote emotional support, reduce feelings of loneliness or isolation, and enhance overall well-being.

Limiting Toxins:

- Minimize exposure to environmental toxins such as pollutants, pesticides, and synthetic chemicals, which can impair immune function and contribute to inflammation and oxidative stress.

Holistic Self-Care:

- Prioritize self-care practices that nurture your physical, emotional, and mental well-being, such as taking regular breaks, practicing gratitude, indulging in hobbies, and seeking professional support when needed.

By incorporating these lifestyle tips into your daily routine, you can maximize the benefits of medicinal mushrooms and enhance your overall health and vitality. Remember that small, consistent actions can lead to significant improvements in well-being over time. Embrace a holistic approach to wellness and let the power of mushrooms support you on your journey to optimal health.

Personalizing Your Mushroom Wellness Routine

As with any wellness journey, personalization is key to success. This section, will help empower you to tailor your mushroom wellness routine to align with your unique goals, preferences, and lifestyle. Whether you're looking to boost immunity, support cognitive function, or enhance emotional well-being, you can craft a personalized approach to mushroom integration that meets your personal needs.

Identify Your Wellness Goals:

- Begin by clarifying your specific health goals and objectives. Are you seeking to improve immune function, enhance cognitive performance, manage stress, or support emotional well-being? Understanding your priorities will guide your mushroom wellness routine.

Choose the Right Mushrooms:

- Select mushroom species that align with your wellness goals and preferences. Research the therapeutic properties of different mushrooms, such as Reishi for relaxation, Lion's Mane for cognitive support, or Cordyceps for energy, and choose accordingly.

Consider Your Lifestyle:

- Take into account your lifestyle, dietary preferences, and daily routines when integrating mushrooms into your wellness regimen. Choose convenient forms of mushroom supplementation, such as capsules, powders, or tinctures, that seamlessly fit into your lifestyle.

Experiment with Different Forms:

- Explore various forms of mushroom products, including supplements, tinctures, teas, extracts, and culinary preparations, to find what works best for you. Experiment with different recipes, dosage forms, and delivery methods to discover your preferred mode of mushroom consumption.

Monitor Your Response:

- Pay attention to how your body responds to mushroom supplementation and adjust your routine accordingly. Keep track of any changes in energy levels, mood, cognitive function, immune function, or overall well-being to determine the effectiveness of your mushroom wellness routine.

Incorporate Mindful Practices:

- Integrate mindfulness practices such as meditation, breathwork, or journaling into your daily routine to enhance the benefits of mushroom supplementation. Cultivating mindfulness can help you stay present, connected, and attuned to your body's needs.

Seek Professional Guidance:

- If you have specific health concerns or medical conditions, consult with a qualified healthcare professional or holistic practitioner for personalized recommendations. They can provide tailored guidance on mushroom selection, dosage, and integration into your wellness routine.

By personalizing your mushroom wellness routine based on

your individual goals, preferences, and lifestyle, you can optimize the benefits of mushroom supplementation. A solid personal integration plan is crucial for each individual. To experience the full benefits of medicinal mushrooms.

Embracing the Power of Mushrooms for Holistic Wellness
Whether enjoyed in culinary creations, supplements, or daily lifestyle practices, mushrooms offer a natural and holistic approach to promoting well-being. Embracing the power of mushrooms nourishes both body and soul, fostering a state of balance and harmony in our lives.

6

Conclusion

As we come to the end of our journey through the world of medicinal mushrooms, it's time to reflect on the profound impact these fungi can have on our health and well-being. Throughout this book, we've explored the diverse benefits of mushrooms such as Reishi, Lion's Mane, Cordyceps, Chaga, Turkey Tail, and Shiitake, learning how they can support immunity, cognitive function, emotional balance, and overall health.

Mushroom medicine reminds us of the interconnectedness of all living beings and the wisdom of the natural world. In cultivating a deeper relationship with mushrooms, we tap into the ancient wisdom of healers and shamans who have long revered these fungi as sacred allies in the journey to wellness.

By understanding the versatility of medicinal mushrooms and incorporating them into our daily lives through culinary creations, supplements, and lifestyle practices, we've unlocked the power of nature's pharmacy to enhance our health on a holistic level. From nourishing broths and savory stir-fries to immune-boosting smoothies and soothing teas, mushrooms have offered us a bounty of delicious and nutritious options to explore.

But our journey doesn't end here—it's just the beginning. As you embark on your own mushroom wellness routine, I encourage you to continue exploring the vast array of mushroom species and integrating them into your daily regimen in a way that aligns with your unique goals and preferences. Whether you're sipping on a Reishi-infused latte to unwind after a long day or incorporating Lion's Mane into your morning routine to sharpen focus and concentration, the possibilities are endless.

So, let us continue to explore, learn, and integrate mushroom medicine into our lives, allowing it to guide us on a journey towards greater mental clarity, emotional balance, and vitality. May the wisdom of mushroom medicine illuminate our path to mental wellness, empowering us to thrive in mind, body, and spirit.

As you navigate your mushroom wellness journey, I invite you to share your experiences and insights with others. Your journey can inspire and empower others to embrace the power of mushrooms for their own lives. I encourage you to leave a review of this book on Amazon, sharing how it has impacted your understanding of medicinal mushrooms and inspired positive changes in your life. Your feedback will help guide others on their own path to wellness and ensure that the transformative potential of mushrooms reaches as many people as possible.

Thank you for joining me on this journey. May you find balance and renewed immunity in the embrace of these wonderful mushrooms. And may you carry forth their wisdom and healing energy into every aspect of your life, nourishing your body, mind, and spirit for years to come.